WALL PILATES WORKOUT FOR WOMEN OVER 60

The Complete Step by Step Guide for Seniors to Achieve Core Strength, Good Posture and Maintain Balance with Less Time

Patricia R. Brickner

TABLE OF CONTENT

INTRODUCTION

These workouts offer several advantages adapted to the special demands of older women. First and foremost, they aim to improve posture and reduce pressure on the spine and joints.

Second, by leveraging the resistance supplied by the wall, these workouts target important muscular areas such as the core, legs, arms, and back, resulting in greater strength and muscle tone.

Understanding the ideas underlying wall Pilates is critical to maximizing its advantages. To begin, stressing good alignment maximizes efficacy while reducing the chance of injury during exercise.

Second, wall Pilates emphasizes activating the core muscles during each action, which promotes stability and strength in the center of the body.

Women over the age of 60 benefit especially from a few specialized workouts.

Wall squats develop the lower body and improve balance, whilst wall push-ups work the chest, shoulders, and arms while putting less strain on the wrists and shoulders than typical floor push-ups.

Wall angels improve shoulder mobility and stability, promote good posture, and lower the chance of shoulder injuries.

Wall planks work the core, shoulders, and legs, increasing strength and stability throughout the body, with variations to suit all fitness levels.

Prioritizing safety is critical when beginning any fitness program, especially for older persons.

Before starting any new fitness plan, consult with a healthcare practitioner, especially if you have pre-existing health issues or concerns.

Starting initially with soft motions and gradually increasing intensity and length is critical for avoiding injury and having a pleasant experience.

Furthermore, listening to your body throughout workouts and changing routines as needed is critical for both safety and enjoyment.

Wall Pilates workouts provide various advantages for women over 60, including increased strength, flexibility, balance, and general well-being. Individuals in this demographic may have a meaningful and productive fitness regimen adapted to their needs and abilities by grasping the fundamentals, integrating suitable activities, and putting safety first.

Chapter 1: Understanding the Benefits of Pilates for Women Over 60

Pilates, a kind of exercise invented by Joseph Pilates in the early twentieth century, has grown in popularity throughout the world due to its multiple health advantages.

Incorporating Pilates into a workout regimen may be especially beneficial for women over 60, supporting general health and improving quality of life.

One of the key advantages of Pilates for women over 60 is increased flexibility and mobility. As we age, our muscles and joints tighten, resulting in diminished flexibility and range of motion.

Pilates focuses on stretching and lengthening muscles to relieve stiffness and enhance mobility, which is essential for retaining independence and avoiding accidents.

Pilates is well known for its ability to strengthen the core muscles. A strong core is necessary for proper posture, balance, and stability, all of which grow more vital as we age.

Pilates, which targets the core muscles, helps women over 60 maintain better posture, lower the risk of falls, and support the spine, enabling a more active and confident lifestyle.

Another key advantage of Pilates for elderly women is its low-impact nature. Pilates, unlike high-impact workouts that can be rough on the joints, is mild but effective, making it appropriate for people who suffer from joint discomfort or arthritis.

It enables women over 60 to engage in physical exercise without exerting undue strain on their bodies, lowering the chance of injury and pain.

Pilates also enhances emotional and physical well-being. Pilates classes, which emphasize regulated movements, breathing, and mindfulness, assist older women improve attention, reduce stress, and increase general mental clarity.

This mind-body link promotes inner serenity and relaxation, which is especially useful for handling daily stressors and improving sleep quality.

Pilates has several benefits for women over 60, including increased flexibility, core strength, joint health, and mental well-being.

 By including Pilates into their workout program, older women may improve their quality of life, preserve independence, and age gracefully and confidently.

Pilates is an excellent kind of exercise for older folks who want to be active, healthy, and vibrant.

Overview of Wall Pilates:
Modifications and Safety Tips

Wall Pilates is a modified version of Pilates that uses a wall for support and stability throughout the movements.

It is especially useful for elders since it gives additional support, making it safer and more accessible to people with restricted movement or balance concerns.

Here's a detailed introduction of wall Pilates, with adjustments and senior-specific safety recommendations.

1. Understanding. Wall Pilates combines classic Pilates movements with the assistance of a wall. The wall acts as a stabilizing force, allowing elderly to execute exercises with improved form

and a lower chance of injury. This Pilates method focuses on increasing strength, flexibility, balance, and posture, all of which are essential for preserving mobility and independence as we age.

2. Modifications for Seniors: a. Props: Using resistance bands, Pilates balls, or foam blocks can help seniors execute exercises more comfortably.

b. Range of Motion Modification: Seniors can change the range of motion in exercises to suit their flexibility and comfort level.
It is advised that you begin with modest motions and progressively increase your range as you gain strength.

c. Chair Support: Seniors can use a chair to increase stability during standing exercises or to provide support while seated against a wall.

d. Reduced Intensity: Seniors must listen to their body and reduce the intensity of their workouts accordingly. Gentle movement and calm breathing are essential.

3. Safety Tips: a. check with a Healthcare Professional: Before beginning an exercise routine, seniors should check with their healthcare practitioner, especially if they have any medical issues or concerns.

b. Warm-Up and Cool Down: A regular warm-up and cool-down program is essential for avoiding injury and preparing the body for activity.

c. *Slow and Controlled Movements:* Seniors should focus on exercising slowly and with control in order to preserve appropriate form and decrease the danger of strains or falls.

d. *Stay Hydrated:* Adequate hydration is critical during activity, particularly for seniors, to avoid weariness and dehydration.

a. *Listen to Your Body:* Seniors should be aware of how their bodies feel during exercise and stop promptly if they encounter pain or discomfort.

Wall Pilates provides seniors with a safe and effective technique to increase strength, flexibility, and balance while reducing the chance of injury.

Seniors may take advantage of the numerous advantages of wall Pilates as part of their overall fitness program by making adaptations and adhering to safety guidelines.

Importance of Proper Warm-up and Cool-down Techniques

Proper warm-up and cool-down practices are critical components of any training plan, especially for women over 60 who participate in wall Pilates sessions.

These preliminary and closing stages are critical to increasing the efficiency of the workout regimen while reducing the danger of damage.

First, a complete warm-up is required to prepare the body for physical activity.

This phase is especially important for women over the age of 60, since their bodies may be more susceptible to stiffness and diminished flexibility.

A warm-up primes the cardiovascular system and improves joint mobility, making it simpler to complete exercises with perfect form.

This is especially important in wall Pilates, where stability and balance are essential components.

Customized warm-up regimens can precisely target regions that may be more vulnerable to injury or strain in older people, such as the lower back or knees.

 Gentle stretches and mobility exercises can help relieve tension and enhance range of motion, resulting in a more seamless transition into the main workout.

Conversely, the cool-down period is also vital for women over 60 who do wall Pilates. It helps the body to gradually return to its resting condition, avoiding sudden decreases in blood pressure and reducing post-exercise muscular discomfort.

Gentle stretching and breathing exercises during this interval encourage relaxation and help in the clearance of metabolic waste products, allowing for speedier healing.

Furthermore, a good cool-down will help reduce the building of lactic acid in the muscles, which can cause soreness and stiffness, especially in older people.

It promotes circulation and lymphatic drainage, which aids the body's natural healing processes, lowering the risk of delayed-onset muscular pain and improving general well-being.

Proper warm-up and cool-down methods are critical for women over 60 who are participating in wall Pilates exercises.

They improve performance, reduce the possibility of injury, and enhance overall physical health and wellness.

By combining these crucial parts into their workout program, people may get the advantages of Pilates while also protecting their bodies' long-term health and vitality.

Chapter 2: Foundational Wall Pilates Exercises

Foundational wall pilates exercises are a mild yet effective technique for women over 60 to enhance strength, flexibility, and balance while putting less load on joints.

These exercises use a wall to offer stability and help with proper alignment, making them appropriate for those with varied degrees of fitness and mobility.

The wall squat is a basic exercise. Standing with your back against the wall, slide down until your knees form a 90-degree angle while keeping your back straight against the wall.

Hold this posture for a few seconds before gradually sliding back up.

This exercise builds strength in the quadriceps, hamstrings, and glutes while also exercising the core muscles for stability.Another useful exercise is the wall roll-down.

Standing with your feet hip-width apart and your back against the wall, gently roll down your spine, one vertebra at a time, until your head, shoulders, and lower back are against the wall.

Engage your core muscles to keep you stable as you roll back up to standing. This exercise increases spinal flexibility and posture while strengthening the abdominal muscles.

Additionally, the wall plank is a fantastic exercise for developing core strength and stability. Start in a plank posture, with your forearms on the wall and your body in a straight line from head to heels.

Hold this posture for as long as you feel comfortable, focusing on using the abdominal and glute muscles to support your body weight.

These basic wall pilates routines may be tailored to different fitness levels and goals.
They offer a safe and accessible alternative for women over 60 to maintain or enhance their physical health while also boosting functional strength and mobility for daily activities.

Incorporating these exercises into your normal workout program will help you have more energy, improve your posture, and feel better overall.

Gentle Wall Stretches to Improve Flexibility and Mobility

Incorporating wall stretches into a Pilates exercise can improve flexibility and mobility in women over 60.

These gentle yet effective stretches use a wall to offer stability while targeting multiple muscle groups, producing improved range of motion and general mobility.

Wall Hip Flexor Stretch: Stand facing the wall, one foot forward, the other stretched behind you.

Place your hands on the wall for support while gradually leaning forward, feeling the stretch in the rear leg's hip flexors.

Hold for 20–30 seconds then swap sides.

Wall Chest Stretch: Stand parallel to the wall with your arm straight out to the side, shoulder height.

Place your hand flat on the wall and gently twist your body away from it, experiencing a stretch in the chest and shoulders. Hold for 20–30 seconds on each side.

Wall Calf Stretch: Stand arm's length away from the wall, with your hands on it for support. Step one foot back and push the heel into the floor, keeping the rear leg straight.

Lean slightly forward to increase the strain in your calf muscle. Hold for 20-30 seconds then swap legs.

Wall Shoulder Stretch: Face the wall and raise one arm straight out in front of you to shoulder height. Place your palm flat on the wall, fingers pointing up.

Gently press into the wall while rotating your body away, experiencing a stretch in your shoulder and chest. Hold for 20 to 30 seconds on each side.

Wall Hamstring Stretch: Sit on the floor with one leg stretched against the wall and the other bent and flat on the ground.
Slowly move your hands down the outstretched leg, reaching for the toes and maintaining your back flat. Hold for 20-30 seconds then swap legs.

Incorporating these mild wall stretches into a Pilates exercise will boost flexibility and mobility, allowing women over 60 to move more easily and comfortably in their everyday lives.

Core Strengthening Exercises for Stability and Balance

As women age, maintaining stability and balance becomes more crucial for their general health and well-being.

Core strengthening exercises, particularly those used in wall Pilates workouts, are a mild yet effective technique for women over 60 to enhance their stability and balance.

Wall Pilates workouts use the assistance of a wall to improve stability while targeting core muscles.

These exercises are low-impact and adaptable to different fitness levels, making them great for older people wishing to develop their strength and balance safely.

One of the main advantages of wall Pilates for women over 60 is that it focuses on core muscles such as the abdominals, obliques, and lower back.

These muscles are essential for maintaining stability and balance, especially as we age and our bodies naturally lose muscular mass.

Women who strengthen their core can improve their posture, lessen their chance of falling, and increase their general stability.

Some frequent core strengthening movements used in wall Pilates sessions for women over 60 include:

Wall Squats: Lean against the wall, feet hip-width apart, and gently drop into a squat posture while keeping your back against the wall. Hold for a few seconds, then gradually return to your starting position.

This workout focuses on the quadriceps, glutes, and core muscles.

Wall Planks: Face the wall and set your hands shoulder-width apart against it at chest height. Step back until the body forms a straight line from head to heels, activating the core muscles.

Maintain this position for 30 seconds to a minute, concentrating on stability and balance.

Wall Bridge: Lying on the floor with feet against the wall and knees bent, lift the hips off the ground while activating the glutes and core muscles.

Hold for a few seconds before gradually lowering back down. This workout focuses on the hamstrings, glutes, and core.

Women over 60 who incorporate these core strengthening exercises into their regimen can enhance their stability, balance, and general quality of life.

Wall Pilates routines, when performed consistently and correctly, provide a safe and effective approach for elderly people to preserve their strength and independence.

Maintaining excellent posture and arm strength is critical for general health and well-being, particularly as we get older.

Wall exercises are an efficient approach for women over 60 to improve their upper bodies without requiring costly equipment.

These exercises work important muscle groups, increasing posture, arm strength, and stability.

To perform wall push-ups, stand a few feet away and face the wall. Place your hands on the wall, a little wider than shoulder width apart and at shoulder height.

Keep your body in a straight line from head to heel. Bend your elbows and lower your chest towards the wall before pushing back to the starting position. Repeat a certain number of times.

Wall Angels: Stand with your back against the wall, feet hip-width apart, and arms by your sides. Slowly lift your arms upward, retaining as much touch with the wall as possible.

As you reach upwards, your arms should make a "Y" shape. Lower your arms back to their starting position, keeping contact with the wall during the exercise.

This exercise improves both shoulder mobility and posture.

Wall Rows: Stand at arm's length, feet shoulder-width apart. Extend your arms and rest your hands against the wall, shoulder height.

Bend your elbows, draw your shoulder blades together, and lift your chest towards the wall while keeping your body straight.
 Pause momentarily at the summit before gently returning to the starting position. This exercise works the muscles in the upper back and improves posture.

Assume a plank stance facing the wall, hands shoulder-width apart and resting on the wall.

Maintain a straight line from head to heels while activating your core and glutes.

Hold this pose for a specific period of time, focusing on perfect alignment and regular breathing. Wall planks increase core strength and general stability.

Incorporating these upper-body strengthening routines into a wall workout regimen can help women over 60 improve their posture, arm strength, and general health and mobility.

Regular use of these exercises can boost confidence and functional independence in everyday tasks.

Chapter 3: Building Strength and Stability

Wall Pilates routines are a unique and effective technique for women over 60 to increase strength and stability while boosting overall fitness.

These workouts use the support of a wall to provide stability and aid, making them suitable for people of any fitness level.

Wall Pilates, which incorporates gentle motions and focused exercises, aims to strengthen the core, improve posture, and improve general balance.

One of the primary advantages of Wall Pilates is its emphasis on developing core strength. As we become older, having a strong core becomes more vital for stability and movement. Wall Pilates routines work the abdominal muscles, obliques, and lower back, promoting core strength and stability.

This not only promotes good posture but also lowers the chance of falls and accidents.

Wall Pilates routines can aid with general stability and balance. Many of the exercises include standing or balancing against a wall, which helps to train the muscles responsible for stability.

This is especially important for elderly persons, who may lose balance owing to age-related reductions in muscular strength and coordination.

Furthermore, Wall Pilates provides a low-impact workout that is easy on the joints. This makes it appropriate for ladies over the age of 60 who may be experiencing joint discomfort or limited mobility.

The wall's supporting nature enables people to complete exercises with perfect form and alignment, lowering their risk of strain or injury.

Incorporating Wall Pilates into your daily training program can result in notable gains in strength, stability, and general fitness.

These workouts, whether done in a group class or on their own at home, provide a safe and effective approach for women over 60 to keep active while also maintaining their health and wellness.

Individuals who practice consistently can gain strength, improve posture, and balance, resulting in a superior quality of life as they age.

Intermediate Wall Pilates Exercises for Strength Development

Intermediate Wall Pilates Exercises for Strength Development provide a focused approach to improving muscular endurance and stability for women over 60.

These exercises make use of the support and resistance given by a wall, allowing for regulated motions that target many muscle groups at once.

Wall Push-Ups: Begin by standing a few feet away from the wall, facing it and holding your hands shoulder-width apart at shoulder level.

Lean forward and place your palms against the wall at shoulder height.

Bend your elbows and lower your chest towards the wall before pushing back to the starting position. This workout strengthens the chest, shoulders, and triceps.

Wall Squats: Stand with your back to the wall and your feet hip-width apart. Lower yourself to a squat position, keeping your knees precisely above your ankles and your back against the wall.

Hold the position for a few seconds, then return to the beginning position. This workout focuses on the quadriceps, hamstrings, and glutes.

Wall Bridge: Lie on your back, feet hip-width apart, knees bent. Place your feet on the wall and elevate your hips toward the ceiling to form a straight line from your knees to your shoulders. Hold the bridge posture for a few seconds, engaging your core and glutes before lowering back down. This exercise builds strength in the lower back, glutes, and hamstrings.

Wall Plank: Start in a plank posture, with your forearms on the floor and your elbows exactly beneath your shoulders.

Walk your feet up the wall, keeping your body in a straight line from head to heels. Hold this stance while working your core and glutes to stay stable.

This workout focuses on the core, shoulders, and lower back.

Incorporating these Intermediate Wall Pilates Exercises into a daily workout program will help women over 60 improve their strength, stability, and general health. Remember to maintain appropriate form and breathing throughout each action to maximize benefits while reducing the chance of injury.

Incorporating Resistance Bands for Added Challenge

Incorporating resistance bands into wall Pilates sessions may provide an additional challenge for women over 60, improving their strength, flexibility, and general fitness.

These routines, particularly targeted for older women, seek to improve posture, boost muscle tone, and promote mobility while reducing joint pain.

Participants can strengthen classic Pilates routines by using resistance bands, which efficiently engage various muscle groups at the same time.

The bands produce resistance throughout the whole range of action, increasing muscular workload and fostering more muscle development and endurance.

Resistance bands may be used in a variety of ways when performing wall Pilates routines.

For example, using bands into workouts like leg pushes against the wall and arm pulls may efficiently tone and build muscles while improving stability and balance.

Resistance bands may be used to add resistance to core-focused workouts like wall planks or wall sits, which aids in the development of a strong and stable core necessary for balance and injury prevention.

Resistance bands are adjustable and portable, making them ideal for at-home exercises and travel. They are readily integrated into a wall Pilates program, letting women over 60 to continue their fitness journey regardless of their location.

Incorporating resistance bands into wall Pilates routines for women over 60 improves strength, flexibility, and overall fitness.

Participants may increase the benefits of their workouts, enhance muscular tone, and live a healthier lifestyle by adding

resistance to classic Pilates routines. With correct instruction and continuous practice, these activities can help older women reach their fitness objectives and reap the numerous advantages of an active lifestyle.

Focus on Lower Body: Leg and Glute Strengthening Techniques.

As women get older, maintaining lower-body strength and mobility becomes increasingly crucial for their general health and independence.

Wall Pilates routines are a safe and effective approach for ladies over 60 to strengthen their legs and glutes without causing excessive stress on their joints.

The Wall Sit is a crucial exercise in Wall Pilates. This workout focuses on the quadriceps, hamstrings, and glutes.

To do a Wall Sit, stand with your back against a strong wall and lower your body until your thighs are parallel to the floor, as if you were sitting in an unseen chair. Hold this position for 30 seconds to a minute, engaging your core and ensuring good alignment.

The Wall Squat is another useful movement. This variant of the standard squat supports the lower back while also activating the leg and glute muscles.

Stand with your feet hip width apart and your back against the wall. Lower yourself into a squat position, keeping your knees in line with your ankles and your weight on your heels. Hold for a few seconds before returning to standing.

Wall Bridges are a great exercise for targeting glutes. Lie on your back, feet flat on the wall and knees bent.

 Lift your hips off the floor, engage your glutes and hamstrings, and then drop them back down. Repeat for 10-15 repetitions, squeezing your glutes at the peak of each action.

Incorporating these Wall Pilates movements into your normal workout program will help women over 60 improve their lower body strength, stability, and balance.

Remember to listen to your body and adjust routines to meet any restrictions or pain.

With persistence and good form, these strategies can help you achieve better overall health and functional fitness as you age.

Chapter 4: Advanced Wall Pilates Techniques

Advanced wall Pilates techniques provide a comprehensive approach to fitness that is particularly designed for ladies over 60.

These exercises use the support of a wall to improve stability, flexibility, and strength while reducing the chance of injury.

These workouts include Pilates concepts to improve posture, core strength, and general body alignment.

The wall roll-down is a crucial technique in which practitioners stand with their backs to the wall and progressively articulate their spine downward, segment by segment, until they attain a forward fold posture. This technique increases spinal mobility and stretches the hamstrings while simultaneously activating the core muscles to keep the body stable against the wall.

Another excellent technique is the wall squat, which works the quadriceps, glutes, and core muscles.

Participants lower into a squat position, keeping their back flat against the wall and their feet hip-width apart. This workout strengthens the lower body and improves balance and posture.

Wall push-ups are an effective way to develop the upper body, particularly the chest, shoulders, and triceps. Push-ups are performed facing the wall with hands shoulder-width apart while maintaining a neutral spine position.

This version puts less strain on the wrists and shoulders than regular floor push-ups.

Wall planks are a demanding core exercise that promotes shoulder stability. Participants face the wall, forearms resting on it and elbows precisely beneath their shoulders.

They elevate their hips to form a straight line from shoulders to heels, using their core muscles, and hold the posture to increase endurance and strength.

Advanced wall Pilates techniques provide a safe and effective workout for women over 60, encouraging functional mobility, muscular strength, and general well-being without the need of sophisticated apparatus or high-impact exercises. These strategies may be adjusted to meet individual fitness levels and goals, giving a diverse approach to preserving health and energy in older years.

Dynamic Wall Pilates Movements for Coordination and Agility

Dynamic Wall Pilates Movements for Coordination and Agility provides a focused method for improving coordination and agility in women over 60.

These specialized workouts make use of a wall to give stability while testing the body's proprioception and balance.

These workouts promote strength, flexibility, and better posture by engaging many muscle groups at the same time through dynamic movements.

Wall-based Pilates workouts for women over 60 emphasize functional motions that mirror everyday tasks including reaching, bending, and lifting. These activities increase coordination by requiring precise control of body movements across many planes of motion.

 Exercises like wall squats with leg lifts or wall push-ups with rotation, for example, require coordination by combining upper and lower body motions while maintaining balance against the wall.

Agility is also an important aspect of Dynamic Wall Pilates movements. These workouts increase response time and general agility by combining short transitions between exercises, as well as speed and rhythm aspects.

Exercises like wall jumps or wall plank variants with leg swings, for example, need quick changes in body posture, which improve agility and proprioception.

The introduction of resistance bands or small equipment like stability balls or foam rollers may offer variety and difficulty to wall Pilates routines.

This equipment may be used in workouts like wall presses with resistance bands or wall squats with a stability ball to increase muscular engagement while improving coordination and agility.

Consistency is key for improving coordination and agility. Women over 60 can benefit from adding Dynamic Wall Pilates Movements to their weekly workout program, progressively increasing the intensity and complexity of the exercises as they develop.

With frequent practice, these workouts can help boost general physical function, minimize the risk of falls, and encourage independence in everyday tasks.

Advanced Core Exercises: Planks, Side Planks, and Variations

Maintaining a strong core is critical for women over 60 in terms of general health and mobility.

Wall Pilates activities are a low-impact yet effective technique to strengthen the core, improve posture, and increase stability.

Among the various exercises offered, planks and side planks, as well as their variants, stand out as advanced core strengtheners that require little movement or equipment.

Planks: Planks are basic core workouts that work numerous muscle groups at once. To do a plank against the wall, stand at arm's length, lean forward, and rest your hands flat against the wall at shoulder height. Walk your feet back until your body is in a straight line from head to heels, using your core muscles to stay stable.

Hold this posture for 30–60 seconds, keeping your core firm and breathing steady.Side planks exercise the obliques and enhance lateral stability.

Begin by standing sideways to the wall, feet hip-width apart. Place one forearm on the wall perpendicular to your body, then step your feet back until your body forms a straight line from head to heels.

Lift your hips off the ground while balancing on your forearms and feet. Hold for 30–60 seconds on each side.

Variations: To add variety and challenge to your wall Pilates routine, try planks and side planks. Try elevating one leg or arm while retaining a plank position to exercise extra stabilizing muscles.

Increase the intensity of side planks by lifting the top leg or reaching the top arm above. To further stimulate the core muscles, try dynamic motions like hip dips or rotations.

Women over 60 may efficiently develop their core muscles, increase balance, and improve overall physical well-being by including advanced core exercises such as planks and side planks into their wall Pilates sessions, without the need for high-impact activities or specialized equipment.

Consistency and perfect technique are essential for maximizing the benefits of these exercises, so begin softly and progressively increase intensity as you gain strength and confidence.

Integrating Pilates Balls and Small Equipment for Intensity

Women over 60 can increase the intensity and efficacy of their training regimens by incorporating small equipment, such as Pilates balls into their Pilates practices.

Individuals may use these props to stimulate specific muscle areas, enhance balance and stability, and vary their routines.

One excellent approach to use Pilates balls is to include them into wall workouts.

For example, placing a Pilates ball between the lower back and the wall during squats can enhance the difficulty by using the core muscles for stability.

Keeping the ball between the thighs during wall sits helps engage the inner thigh muscles, resulting in a more complete lower-body exercise.

Furthermore, Pilates balls may be utilized to provide resistance to standard wall workouts.

Placing the ball below the knees during wall push-ups adds resistance, causing the chest, arms, and core muscles to work harder.

Similarly, holding a Pilates ball between your hands while performing wall presses may efficiently target the triceps and chest muscles.

Small equipment, like resistance bands, can be used in conjunction with Pilates balls to increase the intensity of wall

Pilates workouts. For example, utilizing resistance bands for arm workouts while also exercising the core with a Pilates ball between the lower back and the wall can result in a full-body workout.

Using Pilates balls and small equipment in wall Pilates exercises for women over 60 boosts intensity while also improving safety and lowering the chance of injury.

The wall's support guarantees stability, allowing athletes to focus on appropriate form and technique while testing their muscles with additional resistance.

Including Pilates balls and small equipment in wall Pilates exercises for women over 60 has various advantages, including greater intensity, focused muscle engagement, and improved overall workout efficacy. By imaginatively using these props, people may enjoy a diverse and demanding training regimen that increases strength, stability, and flexibility.

Chapter 5: Functional Movement and Everyday Application

Functional movement refers to workouts and motions that simulate real-life activities and help people improve their strength, flexibility, and mobility for daily chores.

Women over the age of 60 should incorporate functional activities into their workout program to retain independence and general well-being.

Wall Pilates workouts are a low-impact yet effective technique for older women to engage in functional movement exercises that target important muscle groups while emphasizing balance and stability.

One of the key advantages of wall Pilates workouts for ladies over 60 is better posture.
As we age, our posture might suffer owing to factors such as reduced muscular strength and flexibility.

Wall Pilates routines stress perfect alignment and activate the core muscles, which are necessary for healthy posture during workouts and in everyday tasks like standing, walking, and sitting.

Wall Pilates workouts assist in improving functional strength, which is necessary for performing daily duties with ease.

These exercises work muscles across the body, including the legs, arms, and core, which are essential for tasks like lifting groceries, carrying grandkids, and doing housework. Women over 60 who improve their functional strength can lower their chance of injury and retain their independence as they age.

In addition to strength, wall Pilates workouts also focus on flexibility and mobility.

Stretching against the wall increases joint range of motion, making it simpler to accomplish actions such as reaching aloft, bending down to pick up things, and rotating to see behind.

Increased flexibility and mobility improve overall physical comfort while decreasing the chance of stiffness and discomfort associated with aging.

Overall, wall Pilates routines for women over 60 provide a comprehensive approach to functional movement, focusing on important areas such as posture, strength, flexibility, and mobility.

By including these exercises in their fitness program, older women may enhance their quality of life and independence by increasing their capacity to execute daily tasks with confidence and ease.

Translating Wall Pilates Exercises to Daily Activities

Wall Pilates movements provide several advantages for women over 60, including increased flexibility, strength, balance, and general well-being. These exercises, when combined with normal activities, can improve mobility and functioning.

Standing Wall Roll Down: Try this technique while cleaning dishes or brushing your teeth. Stand tall, gradually roll down your spine, then roll back up, activating your core muscles and maintaining stability.

Wall squats may be performed while waiting for the kettle to boil or during commercial breaks. Lean against the wall, squat, and hold, keeping an appropriate posture and working the thigh and glute muscles.

Leg Lifts: While sitting at a desk or watching television, use leg lifts to strengthen your leg muscles. Sit tall, focus your core muscles, and raise one leg at a time, holding momentarily before lowering it with control.

Wall Push-Ups: Incorporate wall push-ups into your regular regimen to build upper-body strength.

Use the kitchen counter or a strong table for support, keeping your hands shoulder-width apart, and executing push-ups against the wall, paying attention to perfect posture, and utilizing your chest and arm muscles.

Pelvic Tilts: Perform pelvic tilts when lying in bed or before waking up in the morning.
Lie on your back, bend your knees, and gradually tilt your pelvis up and down while activating your core muscles and focusing on lower back mobility.

Wall planks can help you strengthen your core muscles and enhance your posture. Lean against the wall at a small angle, activate your core muscles, and hold the position, ensuring a straight line from head to heels.

Perform wall bridges while watching TV or reading to strengthen your hips and glutes.

Lie on your back with your feet against the wall, lift your hips to the ceiling, and hold, activating your glutes and maintaining alignment.

Women over 60 may improve their physical health, increase mobility, and get the advantages of a more active lifestyle by including these Wall Pilates exercises into their regular routines.

Targeting Specific Muscles for
Improved Functionality

As women age, preserving functioning and mobility becomes more vital for their general health and well-being. Wall

Pilates routines provide a targeted method for improving muscular strength, flexibility, and balance that is particularly designed for women over the age of 60.

These workouts, which target particular muscle areas, seek to improve functioning and quality of life.

Wall Pilates routines are known for their ability to efficiently target the core muscles. The core muscles, which include the abdominals, obliques, and lower back, are essential for spine stability and support.

Women over 60 may develop their core muscles by performing exercises such as wall planks, wall squats, and leg lifts against the wall. This improves posture and reduces the chance of falls and accidents.

Wall Pilates routines also highlight the significance of working lower-body muscles such as the glutes, quadriceps, and hamstrings. These muscles are required for everyday tasks such as walking, climbing stairs, and rising from a sitting posture.

Exercises such as wall sits, wall lunges, and wall leg lifts serve to develop these muscles, resulting in increased functioning and mobility.

Upper body movements are another important aspect of Wall Pilates routines for ladies over 60. Strengthening the muscles in the arms, shoulders, and upper back improves not just functional motions but also posture and balance.

Wall push-ups, shoulder presses against the wall, and wall angels are useful workouts for targeting specific muscle areas, allowing women to preserve independence and accomplish everyday duties more comfortably.

Overall, Wall Pilates sessions that target particular muscles help women over 60 enhance their functioning and enjoyment of life.

By strengthening core muscles, lower body muscles, and upper body muscles, these exercises improve posture, balance, and mobility, allowing women to remain active and independent as they age.

Modifications for Common Issues: Arthritis, Osteoporosis, etc.

Wall-based Pilates workouts are a mild but effective approach for women over 60 to strengthen their bodies, increase flexibility, and treat common conditions such as arthritis and osteoporosis.

Individuals may reap the advantages of Pilates while reducing strain and injury risk by altering classic movements to use a wall as support.

Modifications for Arthritis: Wall Pilates movements can be changed to alleviate joint stress in women suffering from arthritis, particularly in the hips, knees, and wrists.
Instead of typical leg lifts or planks on the mat, exercises like wall squats and wall push-ups can give equal benefits while

putting less strain on fragile knees. Gentle stretches against the wall can also enhance range of motion and reduce stiffness.

Modifications for Osteoporosis: Those with osteoporosis should avoid high-impact activities that may increase the risk of fractures.

Wall-based Pilates movements provide a low-impact option while still promoting bone health.

Moves such as wall sits, in which the back is supported against the wall while seated, can assist increase leg and hip strength without causing injury.

Wall push-ups and wall lunges can also help develop muscles and improve balance.

Modifications: Women over 60 may experience diminished mobility, balance difficulties, or muscular weakness.

Wall Pilates routines may be modified to address these difficulties by integrating stability exercises that utilize the wall for support.

Wall angels, in which people stand with their back to the wall and lift their arms aloft while keeping touch with the wall, can assist improve posture and shoulder mobility.

Wall-based Pilates workouts are a diverse and accessible way for women over the age of 60 to enhance their physical health and manage common conditions such as arthritis and osteoporosis.

Individuals may safely and efficiently strengthen their bodies, increase flexibility, and improve their general well-being by adopting simple adaptations to basic Pilates routines.

Chapter 6: Mindfulness and Breathing Techniques

Mindfulness and breathing methods are critical to improving the effectiveness and enjoyment of wall Pilates sessions, particularly for women over 60.

Participants who include mindfulness techniques into their daily routine can strengthen their mind-body connection, increase awareness of their movements, and improve their general well-being.

During wall Pilates workouts, concentrating on breathing methods is critical for maintaining perfect form, engaging core muscles, and increasing stability.

Deep diaphragmatic breathing allows women over 60 to activate their pelvic floor muscles, which are essential for posture and stability, while also aiding relaxation and stress reduction.

Slow, regulated breathing timed with movements helps to maximize the effects of each workout by boosting circulation and increasing oxygen supply to muscles, which is especially advantageous for older persons.

Mindfulness methods like body scanning and proprioceptive awareness may be smoothly integrated into wall Pilates sessions.

Participants can improve their awareness of alignment, muscular engagement, and regions of tension or imbalance by focusing their attention on various body parts and feelings. This increased awareness promotes a stronger link between mind and body, allowing women over 60 to tailor workouts to their own requirements and skills, lowering the risk of injury and improving outcomes.

Mindfulness activities improve mental clarity and attention, allowing participants to completely immerse themselves in the present moment throughout wall Pilates sessions.

This increased attention promotes awareness, reduces distractions, and allows women over 60 to completely participate with each movement and breath.

As a consequence, people may get more happiness and fulfillment out of their workouts, while simultaneously reaping the physical and emotional advantages of Pilates.

Incorporating mindfulness and breathing methods into wall Pilates exercises for women over 60 improves the effectiveness, safety, and pleasure of their training session.

Participants who practice mindfulness and learn breathing methods may improve their Pilates practice, enhance overall well-being, and empower themselves to live active and satisfying lives.

Importance of Mind-Body Connection in Pilates Practice

The mind-body link is crucial to Pilates practice, particularly for women over 60 who perform wall Pilates.

This comprehensive technique stresses the combination of physical activity, mental attention, and awareness.
Individuals can get a variety of advantages from fostering this connection, including improved general well-being.

Women over the age of 60 must maintain their strength, flexibility, and balance in order to age well.

Wall Pilates exercises create a supportive setting in which participants may use the resistance offered by the wall to improve their movements. Individuals can reduce their risk of injury by developing a better knowledge of their body's capabilities and limits through mindful participation.

The mind-body link in Pilates promotes mindfulness and presence throughout the exercise.

Women over the age of 60 may find this especially useful since it allows them to tune into their body, listen to their needs, and modify the exercises as needed.

This increased awareness encourages self-care and compassion, enabling people to move in ways that are both healthy and sustainable.

In addition to the physical advantages, Pilates' mind-body connection promotes mental well-being.

As women face the obstacles of aging, preserving cognitive function and emotional resilience becomes critical.

Pilates provides a space for people to relieve tension, relax, and gain mental clarity. Participants may quiet their minds by coordinating their breath and movement, producing a sensation of serenity and inner peace.

Pilates mind-body connection has an impact on daily living outside of the class. Women over the age of 60 who incorporate Pilates concepts into their daily routines may see improvements in their posture, energy levels, and mobility.

These benefits enable people to participate more completely in their daily activities, encouraging independence and vitality.

The significance of the mind-body link in Pilates cannot be emphasized, particularly for women over 60 who participate in wall Pilates sessions.

Individuals can improve their overall well-being by combining physical activity with mental attention and awareness, which promotes strength, flexibility, balance, mindfulness, and mental resilience.

This comprehensive method promotes healthy aging, allowing women to thrive on and off the mat.

Incorporating Breathing Techniques for Stress Relief and Relaxation

Incorporating mindful breathing methods with wall exercises can greatly improve stress release and relaxation, particularly for women over 60.

As people age, prioritizing mental and physical well-being becomes increasingly important, and combining breathing practices with Pilates against a wall provides a comprehensive method for accomplishing these goals.

Stress release through regulated breathing is critical for general health, and combining it with Pilates movements increases its effectiveness.

During wall Pilates workouts, concentrating on deep inhalations and gentle exhalations activates the parasympathetic nervous system, increasing tranquility and lowering stress.

This mindful breathing method encourages users to time their breath with each exercise, resulting in a stronger mind-body connection.

Incorporating breathing methods into wall Pilates sessions also helps with relaxation by increasing muscular oxygenation and circulation.

Women over the age of 60 may feel stiffness and limited flexibility; appropriate breathing methods can allow smoother movements and relieve muscular tension, resulting in a more pleasurable and successful training experience.

Furthermore, focused breathing throughout wall Pilates exercises improves attention and awareness.

By focusing on the breath, participants may stay present in the moment, allowing them to fully engage in each activity and gain the most benefits.

This mindfulness part of the practice not only helps with stress reduction, but it also fosters a sense of inner calm and wellbeing.

Including breathing methods into wall Pilates sessions enables women over 60 to take charge of their health and fitness journeys.

By including mindful breathing into their workout regimen, people can improve mental clarity, reduce anxiety, and increase overall vitality.

Incorporating breathing methods into wall Pilates sessions for women over 60 provides a comprehensive approach to stress reduction and relaxation.

Participants may have a refreshing and rewarding workout experience that feeds both body and mind by focusing on mindful breathing in addition to physical activity.

Mindfulness Practices to Enhance
Overall Well-being

Mindfulness techniques can dramatically improve overall well-being, particularly when combined with wall pilates routines for women over 60.

These activities develop a stronger connection between mind and body, increasing awareness and presence during exercise.

Individuals who focus on the present moment without judgment can enhance their physical health and mental clarity.

During wall Pilates workouts, mindfulness methods like breath awareness are essential. Participants who intentionally observe their breath may modulate their inhales and exhales, encouraging relaxation and lowering stress levels. This focused breathing also aids in the proper engagement of the core muscles, hence increasing the workout's advantages.

Mindfulness also helps women over the age of 60 to connect with their bodies and pay attention to their bodily experiences.
Participants can avoid injuries and improve their training experience by paying attention to minor indicators like muscle strain or joint soreness.

Mindfulness activities go beyond the physical part of wall pilates. Women over the age of 60 can improve their emotional well-being by practicing mindfulness.

Acknowledging and accepting thoughts and feelings without being attached to them promotes inner calm and resilience.

Mindfulness can boost cognitive performance and mental agility in older persons.
Women over 60 can improve their mental health by including mindfulness activities like focused attention and body scanning into their pilates sessions.

Integrating mindfulness techniques with wall pilates sessions for women over 60 provides a comprehensive approach to improving overall health.

Mindfulness enhances physical health, emotional resilience, and cognitive vigor by cultivating a stronger link between mind and body, eventually encouraging individuals to live better and more rewarding lives.

Chapter 7: Creating Your Personalized Wall Pilates Routine

Pilates, a low-impact fitness program that emphasizes core strength, flexibility, and total body awareness, is widely regarded as having a transforming effect on physical well-being, particularly among women over the age of 60.

Integrating wall exercises into your Pilates regimen can boost its effectiveness by utilizing the support and resistance offered by vertical surfaces.

Creating a personalized wall Pilates program based on the individual requirements and skills of women in this age bracket offers a safe, effective, and fun workout.

Begin your tailored program with a mild warm-up to prepare the body for activity while reducing the chance of injury.

Include dynamic stretches and mobility exercises that target the spine, hips, shoulders, and ankles to improve flexibility and range of motion.

During standing stretches, lean against the wall to help extend the muscles and release tension.

Move on to strengthening exercises for the core, legs, arms, and back. Wall squats, in which you lean against a wall with your feet hip-width apart and drop into a sitting posture, work the quadriceps, glutes, and core muscles while reducing stress on the knees and lower back. Modified push-ups with hands placed on the wall at shoulder height give a good upper-body workout without putting too much pressure on the wrists or shoulders.

Integrate balance and stability exercises into your regimen to improve coordination and proprioception, which are essential for preserving mobility and avoiding falls as we age.

 Wall-supported single-leg stands or leg lifts test stability while offering a safe environment for exploration and advancement.

Finish your wall Pilates workout with a series of calming stretches and deep breathing exercises to aid in relaxation and recuperation. Use the wall as support during sitting or laying stretches to get a deeper stretch while maintaining appropriate alignment and posture.

Create a personalized wall Pilates practice adapted to the individual requirements and capabilities of women over 60 to get the various advantages of this flexible workout modality while reducing the risk of injury and enhancing enjoyment and fulfillment.

Designing a Customized Pilates Routine Based on Individual Needs

Creating a Pilates routine adapted to the specific needs of women over 60 entails a planned combination of exercises that emphasize flexibility, strength, balance, and posture.

Wall Pilates movements can be especially effective in this regimen since they provide support and stability while addressing many muscle groups.

To begin, analyze the individual's current fitness level as well as any specific concerns or limits.

This evaluation assists in developing a routine that efficiently fulfills their requirements while assuring safety and progressive advancement.

Begin with moderate warm-up activities like shoulder rolls and neck stretches to prepare your body for more difficult actions.

Wall-assisted stretches, such as calf stretches and chest openers, can increase flexibility and relieve the stiffness that comes with aging.

Next, incorporating wall squats and wall sits into the practice helps to develop the lower body, especially the quadriceps, hamstrings, and glutes, while also increasing balance and stability.

These exercises may be changed to fit the individual's skills, progressively increasing the time or depth of the motions as they advance.

Incorporating exercises like wall planks and wall push-ups into your core strengthening routine strengthens the abdominal muscles, obliques, and upper body while using the wall as support.

These motions not only strengthen the core, but they also improve general stability and posture, which is essential for maintaining balance and avoiding falls.

Integrating wall-assisted leg lifts and knee lifts stimulates the hip flexors, thighs, and abdominal muscles, which helps to improve mobility and functional movement patterns.

Cooldown stretches against the wall, which target areas of stiffness or discomfort, increase relaxation and flexibility while lowering the risk of muscular soreness.

Throughout the personalized program, attention should be made on good breathing methods and conscious movement to ensure a holistic approach to physical well-being.

Regular changes and tweaks to the program based on success and individual input are required to maximize outcomes and sustain motivation.

Individuals may enhance their strength, flexibility, balance, and overall well-being by adapting a Pilates practice that includes wall exercises to the unique

needs of women over 60, allowing them
to live active and satisfying lives.

Setting Realistic Goals and Tracking Progress Over Time

Setting realistic objectives and evaluating progress over time are critical components of any fitness program, particularly for women over 60 who participate in wall Pilates routines.

Setting reasonable targets ensures that efforts are focused and sustainable, encouraging general well-being and success.

First and foremost, while creating goals, individual talents and constraints must be considered. For women over 60, this may entail taking into consideration current strength, flexibility, and any medical issues.

Realistic goals might include strengthening core strength, flexibility, and balance, all of which are essential to Pilates.

Goals must be precise, measurable, achievable, relevant, and time-bound (SMART). For example, a specific aim may be to hold a plank against the wall for 30 seconds, which can be measured by timing each attempt.

This aim is realistic for many women over 60 and related to core strength development, with a time frame for growth.

Once goals have been defined, tracking progress is critical for keeping motivated and adapting as needed. Keeping a workout log or using fitness monitoring apps may help you measure your gains in strength, flexibility, and endurance over time. Progress in wall Pilates workouts may be seen as increased stability during exercises, improved posture, or the capacity to maintain hard poses for extended periods of time.

Regularly reassessing objectives and changing them depending on progress is essential for keeping on track.

Women over 60 who participate in wall Pilates workouts may discover that their initial goals become simpler to reach or that they are ready to push themselves farther.

Individuals may continue to push their limitations without burning out or injuring themselves by continually reviewing and modifying their goals.

Setting reasonable objectives and evaluating progress over time are critical for women over 60 who engage in wall Pilates sessions.

Individuals may get the full advantages of Pilates while remaining motivated and well-balanced by setting reasonable goals, reviewing progress, and adapting as required.

*Tips for Consistency and Motivation
in Home Practice*

Home-based exercises, particularly wall Pilates routines, are a handy and efficient approach for women over 60 to improve their strength, flexibility, and general health. However, remaining consistent and motivated might be difficult.

Below are some guide to help you stay motivated

1. Set realistic goals: Create attainable goals based on your exercise level and health objectives. Having defined goals, whether they be to improve balance, core strength, or flexibility, can help you stay focused and motivated.

2. Create a Routine: Plan regular sessions for your wall Pilates routines.

Consistency is essential for noticing results and receiving the advantages of your practice. Set aside a certain period each day or week to focus your workout program.

3. *Create a Dedicated Space:* Set aside a separate section of your home for Pilates practice. Keep it clutter-free and stocked with essential props such as a yoga mat, resistance bands, and a firm chair or wall for support during workouts.

4. *range is Key:* Mix up your workouts by combining a range of Pilates movements that target various muscle regions. This not only avoids boredom but also assures a well-rounded workout regimen that pushes your body in a variety of ways.

5. *Listen to Your Body:* Notice how your body feels during and after each session. Respect your boundaries and don't push yourself too hard, especially if you're new to Pilates or have physical restrictions. Exercises can be modified as needed to meet your comfort level.

6. *Stay Motivated:* Find motivation to keep you going on your fitness adventure. This might be accomplished through uplifting music, inspiring phrases, or by joining a supportive network of like-minded people, either online or in person.

7. *Celebrate Progress:* Recognize and celebrate your accomplishments along the road, no matter how minor they appear. Progress in fitness takes time, so be patient with yourself and enjoy your accomplishments.

By implementing these suggestions into your home-based wall Pilates practice, you may increase consistency and motivation, resulting in better physical health and general well-being.

Chapter 8: Safety Tips and Precautions

Wall Pilates workouts provide various advantages for women over 60, including better posture, flexibility, and core strength.

However, prioritizing safety is critical to avoiding accidents and ensuring a successful workout. Here are some important safety guidelines to remember:

Check with a Healthcare Professional: Before beginning any new fitness routine, especially if you have pre-existing health ailments or concerns, you should check with your healthcare practitioner.

They may provide specialized advice and guarantee that Wall Pilates is appropriate for your specific requirements.

Warm-Up Begin each session with a mild warm-up to get your body ready for exercise.

This might involve modest aerobic exercises like walking or marching in place, as well as dynamic stretches to release muscles and joints.

Maintain Proper Form: To minimize strain or injury, keep your form consistent throughout the workout.

Listen to your instructor's signals and focus on alignment, especially while utilizing the wall for support during exercises.

Start Slowly and Progress Gradually: If you're new to Pilates or haven't worked out in a while, begin with beginner-friendly motions and gradually raise the intensity as your strength and confidence grow.

Avoid going beyond limit, especially if it's your first timeListen to your body. During the workout, make sure to comply with the effect your body gives

If you feel pain or discomfort, stop immediately and review your form. It is natural to feel pushed while exercising, but intense or continuous discomfort indicates that something is wrong.

Stay Hydrated: Drink water before, during, and after your workout to maintain hydration. Dehydration can impair performance and raise your risk of injury, so refill fluids on a regular basis.

Invest in High-Quality Pilates Equipment: To improve safety and comfort during Wall Pilates sessions, consider purchasing a non-slip yoga mat and supportive footwear.

Women over the age of 60 can benefit from wall Pilates while reducing their risk of injury by following these safety recommendations and measures.

Remember to listen to your body, emphasize appropriate form, and seek advice from a healthcare expert if you have any concerns.

Pilates, when approached correctly, can be a profitable and fun workout for women of all ages.

Understanding Limitations and Listening to Your Body

Understanding one's body's limitations is critical, especially when participating in physical activities like wall exercises, which are specifically designed for women over 60.

As people age, their bodies suffer a variety of changes, including decreased flexibility, strength, and balance. Thus, it is critical to approach such workouts with attention and adaptation.

Listening to your body is essential during wall pilates sessions. It entails being sensitive to cues such as discomfort, pain, and weariness.

Pushing past these signals may result in injury or strain, which is detrimental to the purpose of enhancing health and fitness. Instead, participants should focus on good form and alignment while respecting their body's limitations.

Modifying exercises to meet individual needs is another important component of wall pilates for older women.

This might include employing supports like blocks or straps to improve stability or limiting the range of motion to avoid overexertion. Participants may reap the advantages of pilates while being safe by adapting the practice to their personal requirements and limits.

Maintaining a steady and progressive technique is also important in wall pilates for older ladies. It's completely fine if you're making slower progress than younger people.

Small triumphs should be celebrated, and the goal should be to gradually improve general strength, flexibility, and balance.

In addition to physical modifications, mental attitude is critical to success with wall pilates. Cultivating an attitude of patience, self-compassion, and resilience can help people overcome obstacles and disappointments on their fitness journeys.

Overall, wall pilates routines for women over 60 rely on recognizing one's own limitations and listening to one's body. Participants may reap the advantages of pilates while respecting their bodies' demands and capacities by embracing adaptation, adjustment, and patience.

Consulting with a Healthcare Professional Before Starting

Before starting a new fitness plan, especially one developed for a specific group, such as women over 60, consult with a healthcare practitioner.

This phase is highly important in Wall Pilates exercises since it may enhance joint health, balance, and overall well-being.

Before beginning Wall Pilates exercises, speak with a healthcare professional to ensure you receive personalized coaching based on your medical history, current health status, and any pre-existing conditions.

This proactive method helps to discover any potential risks or contraindications that must be addressed before beginning the exercise program.

For women over the age of 60, bone density, joint flexibility, and muscle strength become more important.

Wall Pilates workouts can provide a variety of benefits, including improved posture, core strength, and balance, which are especially useful to seniors.

However, in order to prevent harm and maximize effectiveness, these exercises must be customized to each individual's specific needs and limitations.

Healthcare professionals may provide valuable insights and recommendations for alterations or alternate exercises that are more appropriate for the individual's talents and goals. They may also provide advice on proper technique, breathing patterns, and gradual growth to minimize overtraining and improve long-term sustainability.

Speaking with a healthcare specialist fosters a collaborative approach to health and fitness, allowing people to make informed decisions about their own health.

It encourages open communication and fosters a supportive environment in which questions and concerns may be appropriately addressed.

Before beginning Wall Pilates exercises, women over 60 should consult with a healthcare professional to ensure a safe, successful, and tailored approach to their fitness journey. Individuals who take this proactive approach may be able to optimize their experience and reap the full benefits of this specific training routine while limiting potential risks.

*Creating a Safe Exercise
Environment: Proper Equipment and
Space Arrangement*

Creating a safe training setting is critical, especially for women over 60 who participate in wall Pilates routines. Proper equipment and space organization are critical in maintaining safety and optimizing the advantages of the training regimen.

To begin, while designing the training environment, select a clear, clutter-free place with plenty of freedom to move around.

Remove any impediments or risks that may cause a trip or fall. Additionally, ensure that the floor is clean and non-slip to avoid mishaps, particularly during balancing exercises.

Invest on high-quality Pilates equipment, such as resistance bands, stability balls, and foam rollers.
These gadgets not only make the workout more effective, but they also give support and stability, which is especially important for older persons.

To avoid accidents or injuries, ensure that the equipment is in excellent working order and has been regularly maintained.

Proper space arrangement is also vital for safety during wall Pilates practices. Position any wall-mounted equipment, such as resistance bands or wall bars, securely and at a height that is easy to reach without effort.

Place mirrors strategically to allow participants to check their form and alignment while exercising.

Also, consider the illumination in the workout area. Ample natural light or well-placed artificial lighting can increase visibility and lower the risk of an accident, particularly for elderly persons with impaired eyesight.

Provide appropriate ventilation to provide a comfortable training atmosphere. Proper airflow may reduce overheating and improve breathing during workouts, increasing overall safety and pleasure.

It is critical to offer clear instructions and assistance for utilizing the equipment and executing exercises properly. Encourage participants to listen to their bodies and adjust their motions as necessary to minimize strain or damage.

Women over the age of 60 may enjoy wall Pilates workouts safely and successfully by focusing adequate equipment and space layout, which improves their strength, flexibility, and general health.

CONCLUSION

Wall Pilates routines are a very useful and accessible training plan for ladies over 60.

These workouts, which use a combination of mild yet effective motions, give several physical and mental health advantages that are specifically designed for this group.

To begin, wall Pilates exercises increase strength and flexibility, which helps address typical age-related concerns including muscle weakness and joint stiffness.

Participants may use the wall as support to do exercises that target important muscle areas such as the core, legs, and arms, therefore improving overall strength and stability. This is critical for retaining independence and lowering the risk of falls, which is especially significant as people age.

Second, wall Pilates workouts stress good alignment and posture, which are critical for avoiding accidents and maintaining long-term spinal health.

Many older persons suffer from back pain and postural concerns, and these exercises can help improve symptoms by strengthening the muscles that support the spine and promoting better alignment during everyday tasks.

Wall Pilates routines involve mindfulness and relaxation techniques, which are helpful to both physical and mental health. The emphasis on regulated breathing and focused movement reduces tension and increases general relaxation, resulting in a sensation of serenity and mental clarity.

Wall Pilates routines are flexible to different fitness levels and may be tailored to specific health issues or limits. This makes them appropriate for women over 60 who have various degrees of fitness or mobility, offering inclusion and accessibility.

Overall, wall Pilates routines provide a comprehensive approach to fitness and well-being for women over 60.

These exercises, which target strength, flexibility, posture, and mindfulness, help to improve physical health, decrease stress, and improve quality of life. Incorporating wall Pilates into a daily fitness program can help older women stay active and healthy far into their retirement years.

THANK YOU PAGE

Thank you for selecting this book. Your support is really appreciated. Similarly, I am grateful for the purchase of this book. Your input is valuable; please share your ideas in a review. It serves as a reference for future improvements. Enjoy reading and utilizing it!

Workout planner to help track progress and improvements

Workout Planner to Track progress

	EXERCISE	GOAL
MON DAY		
TUES DAY		
WEDNES DAY		
THURS DAY		
FRI DAY		
SAT DAY		

Workout Planner to Track progress

	EXERCISE	GOAL
MON DAY		
TUES DAY		
WEDNES DAY		
THURS DAY		
FRI DAY		
SAT DAY		

Workout Planner to Track progress

	EXERCISE	GOAL
MON DAY		
TUES DAY		
WEDNES DAY		
THURS DAY		
FRI DAY		
SAT DAY		

Workout Planner to Track progress

	EXERCISE	GOAL
MON DAY		
TUES DAY		
WEDNES DAY		
THURS DAY		
FRI DAY		
SAT DAY		

Workout Planner to Track progress

	EXERCISE	GOAL
MON DAY		
TUES DAY		
WEDNES DAY		
THURS DAY		
FRI DAY		
SAT DAY		

Workout Planner to Track progress

	EXERCISE	GOAL
MON DAY		
TUES DAY		
WEDNES DAY		
THURS DAY		
FRI DAY		
SAT DAY		

Workout Planner to Track progress

	EXERCISE	GOAL
MON DAY		
TUES DAY		
WEDNES DAY		
THURS DAY		
FRI DAY		
SAT DAY		

Workout Planner to Track progress

	EXERCISE	GOAL
MON DAY		
TUES DAY		
WEDNES DAY		
THURS DAY		
FRI DAY		
SAT DAY		

Workout Planner to Track progress

	EXERCISE	GOAL
MON DAY		
TUES DAY		
WEDNES DAY		
THURS DAY		
FRI DAY		
SAT DAY		

Workout Planner to Track progress

	EXERCISE	GOAL
MON DAY		
TUES DAY		
WEDNES DAY		
THURS DAY		
FRI DAY		
SAT DAY		

Workout Planner to Track progress

	EXERCISE	GOAL
MONDAY		
TUESDAY		
WEDNESDAY		
THURSDAY		
FRIDAY		
SATDAY		

Workout Planner to Track progress

	EXERCISE	GOAL
MON DAY		
TUES DAY		
WEDNES DAY		
THURS DAY		
FRI DAY		
SAT DAY		

Workout Planner to Track progress

	EXERCISE	GOAL
MON DAY		
TUES DAY		
WEDNES DAY		
THURS DAY		
FRI DAY		
SAT DAY		

Workout Planner to Track progress

	EXERCISE	GOAL
MON DAY		
TUES DAY		
WEDNES DAY		
THURS DAY		
FRI DAY		
SAT DAY		

Workout Planner to Track progress

	EXERCISE	GOAL
MON DAY		
TUES DAY		
WEDNES DAY		
THURS DAY		
FRI DAY		
SAT DAY		

Workout Planner to Track progress

	EXERCISE	GOAL
MON DAY		
TUES DAY		
WEDNES DAY		
THURS DAY		
FRI DAY		
SAT DAY		

Workout Planner to Track progress

	EXERCISE	GOAL
MON DAY		
TUES DAY		
WEDNES DAY		
THURS DAY		
FRI DAY		
SAT DAY		

Workout Planner to Track progress

	EXERCISE	GOAL
MON DAY		
TUES DAY		
WEDNES DAY		
THURS DAY		
FRI DAY		
SAT DAY		

Workout Planner to Track progress

	EXERCISE	GOAL
MON DAY		
TUES DAY		
WEDNES DAY		
THURS DAY		
FRI DAY		
SAT DAY		

Workout Planner to Track progress

	EXERCISE	GOAL
MON DAY		
TUES DAY		
WEDNES DAY		
THURS DAY		
FRI DAY		
SAT DAY		

Workout Planner to Track progress

	EXERCISE	GOAL
MON DAY		
TUES DAY		
WEDNES DAY		
THURS DAY		
FRI DAY		
SAT DAY		

Workout Planner to Track progress

	EXERCISE	GOAL
MON DAY		
TUES DAY		
WEDNES DAY		
THURS DAY		
FRI DAY		
SAT DAY		

Workout Planner to Track progress

	EXERCISE	GOAL
MON DAY		
TUES DAY		
WEDNES DAY		
THURS DAY		
FRI DAY		
SAT DAY		

Workout Planner to Track progress

	EXERCISE	GOAL
MON DAY		
TUES DAY		
WEDNES DAY		
THURS DAY		
FRI DAY		
SAT DAY		

Workout Planner to Track progress

	EXERCISE	GOAL
MON DAY		
TUES DAY		
WEDNES DAY		
THURS DAY		
FRI DAY		
SAT DAY		

Workout Planner to Track progress

	EXERCISE	GOAL
MON DAY		
TUES DAY		
WEDNES DAY		
THURS DAY		
FRI DAY		
SAT DAY		

Workout Planner to Track progress

	EXERCISE	GOAL
MONDAY		
TUESDAY		
WEDNESDAY		
THURSDAY		
FRIDAY		
SATDAY		

Workout Planner to Track progress

	EXERCISE	GOAL
MON DAY		
TUES DAY		
WEDNES DAY		
THURS DAY		
FRI DAY		
SAT DAY		

Workout Planner to Track progress

	EXERCISE	GOAL
MON DAY		
TUES DAY		
WEDNES DAY		
THURS DAY		
FRI DAY		
SAT DAY		

Workout Planner to Track progress

	EXERCISE	GOAL
MON DAY		
TUES DAY		
WEDNES DAY		
THURS DAY		
FRI DAY		
SAT DAY		

Workout Planner to Track progress

	EXERCISE	GOAL
MONDAY		
TUESDAY		
WEDNESDAY		
THURSDAY		
FRIDAY		
SATDAY		

Workout Planner to Track progress

	EXERCISE	GOAL
MON DAY		
TUES DAY		
WEDNES DAY		
THURS DAY		
FRI DAY		
SAT DAY		

Workout Planner to Track progress

	EXERCISE	GOAL
MON DAY		
TUES DAY		
WEDNES DAY		
THURS DAY		
FRI DAY		
SAT DAY		

Workout Planner to Track progress

	EXERCISE	GOAL
MONDAY		
TUESDAY		
WEDNESDAY		
THURSDAY		
FRIDAY		
SATURDAY		

Workout Planner to Track progress

	EXERCISE	GOAL
MON DAY		
TUES DAY		
WEDNES DAY		
THURS DAY		
FRI DAY		
SAT DAY		

Workout Planner to Track progress

	EXERCISE	GOAL
MON DAY		
TUES DAY		
WEDNES DAY		
THURS DAY		
FRI DAY		
SAT DAY		

Workout Planner to Track progress

	EXERCISE	GOAL
MON DAY		
TUES DAY		
WEDNES DAY		
THURS DAY		
FRI DAY		
SAT DAY		

Workout Planner to Track progress

	EXERCISE	GOAL
MON DAY		
TUES DAY		
WEDNES DAY		
THURS DAY		
FRI DAY		
SAT DAY		

Workout Planner to Track progress

	EXERCISE	GOAL
MONDAY		
TUESDAY		
WEDNESDAY		
THURSDAY		
FRIDAY		
SATDAY		

Workout Planner to Track progress

	EXERCISE	GOAL
MON DAY		
TUES DAY		
WEDNES DAY		
THURS DAY		
FRI DAY		
SAT DAY		

Workout Planner to Track progress

	EXERCISE	GOAL
MON DAY		
TUES DAY		
WEDNES DAY		
THURS DAY		
FRI DAY		
SAT DAY		

Workout Planner to Track progress

	EXERCISE	GOAL
MON DAY		
TUES DAY		
WEDNES DAY		
THURS DAY		
FRI DAY		
SAT DAY		

Workout Planner to Track progress

	EXERCISE	GOAL
MON DAY		
TUES DAY		
WEDNES DAY		
THURS DAY		
FRI DAY		
SAT DAY		

Workout Planner to Track progress

	EXERCISE	GOAL
MON DAY		
TUES DAY		
WEDNES DAY		
THURS DAY		
FRI DAY		
SAT DAY		

Workout Planner to Track progress

	EXERCISE	GOAL
MON DAY		
TUES DAY		
WEDNES DAY		
THURS DAY		
FRI DAY		
SAT DAY		

Workout Planner to Track progress

	EXERCISE	GOAL
MONDAY		
TUESDAY		
WEDNESDAY		
THURSDAY		
FRIDAY		
SATDAY		

Workout Planner to Track progress

	EXERCISE	GOAL
MON DAY		
TUES DAY		
WEDNES DAY		
THURS DAY		
FRI DAY		
SAT DAY		

Workout Planner to Track progress

	EXERCISE	GOAL
MON DAY		
TUES DAY		
WEDNES DAY		
THURS DAY		
FRI DAY		
SAT DAY		

Workout Planner to Track progress

	EXERCISE	GOAL
MON DAY		
TUES DAY		
WEDNES DAY		
THURS DAY		
FRI DAY		
SAT DAY		

Workout Planner to Track progress

	EXERCISE	GOAL
MON DAY		
TUES DAY		
WEDNES DAY		
THURS DAY		
FRI DAY		
SAT DAY		

Workout Planner to Track progress

	EXERCISE	GOAL
MON DAY		
TUES DAY		
WEDNES DAY		
THURS DAY		
FRI DAY		
SAT DAY